YOGA
AN ADULT
COLORING BOOK

Relaxing Coloring Pages for Stress Relief and Mindfulness with Yoga, Mandala, and Chakra Inspired Designs

*** Color Test Page At End of Book*

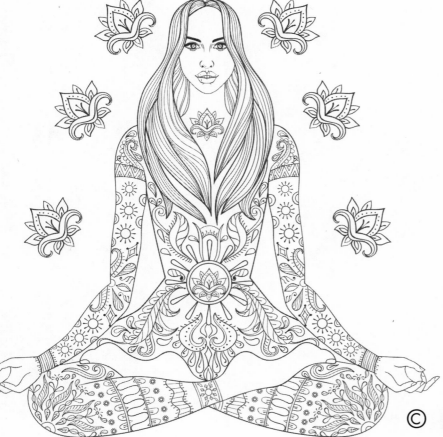

© 2021 CNandJ.com

The back of each coloring page has a black backing to protect against bleeding when using markers or ink pens.

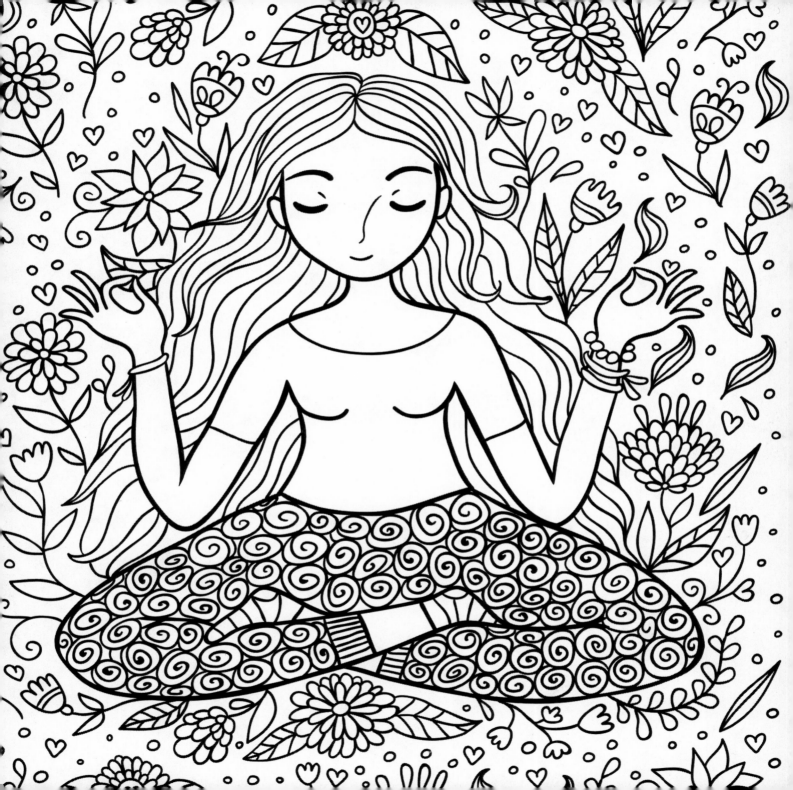

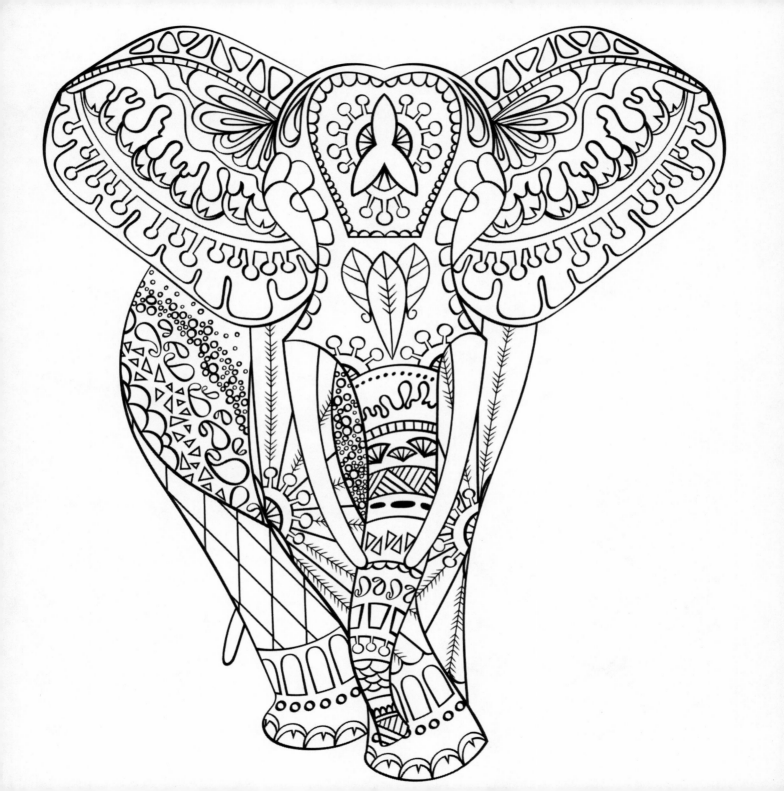

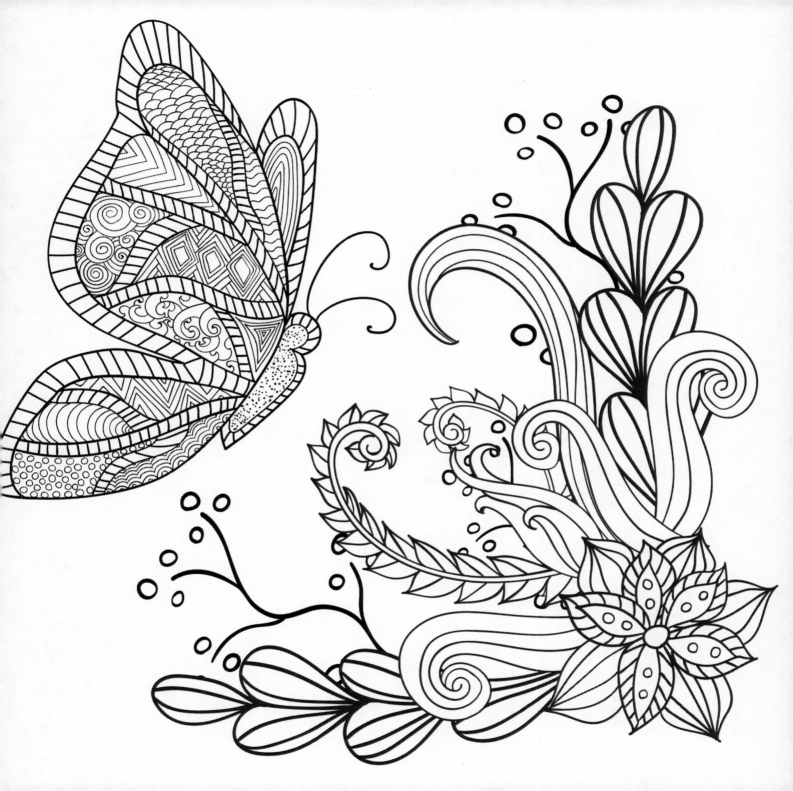

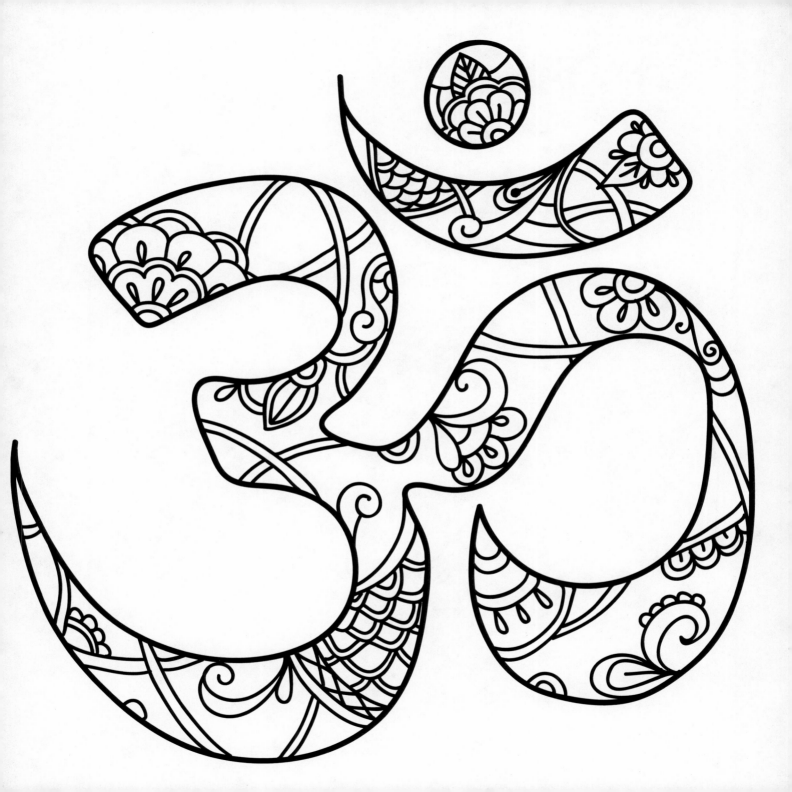

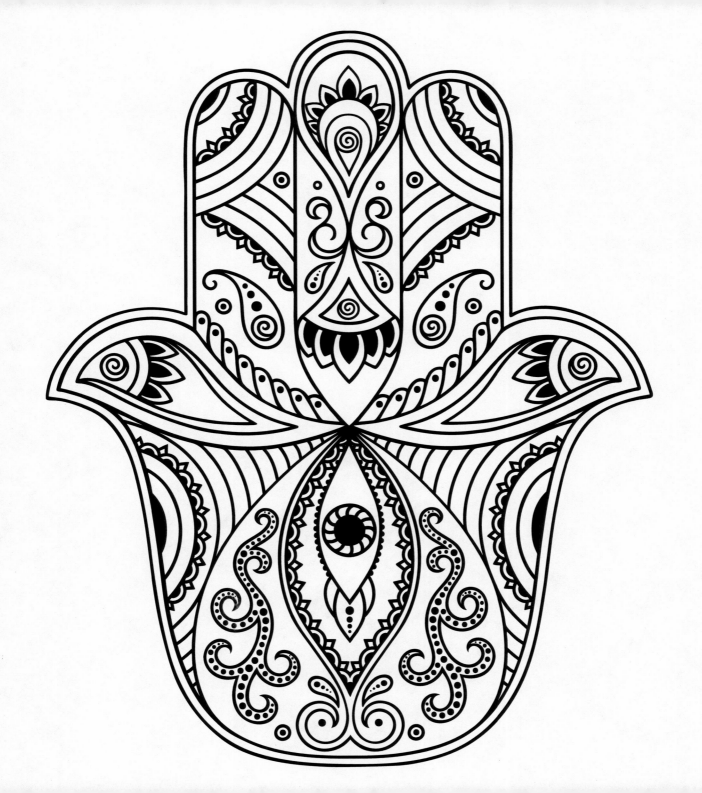

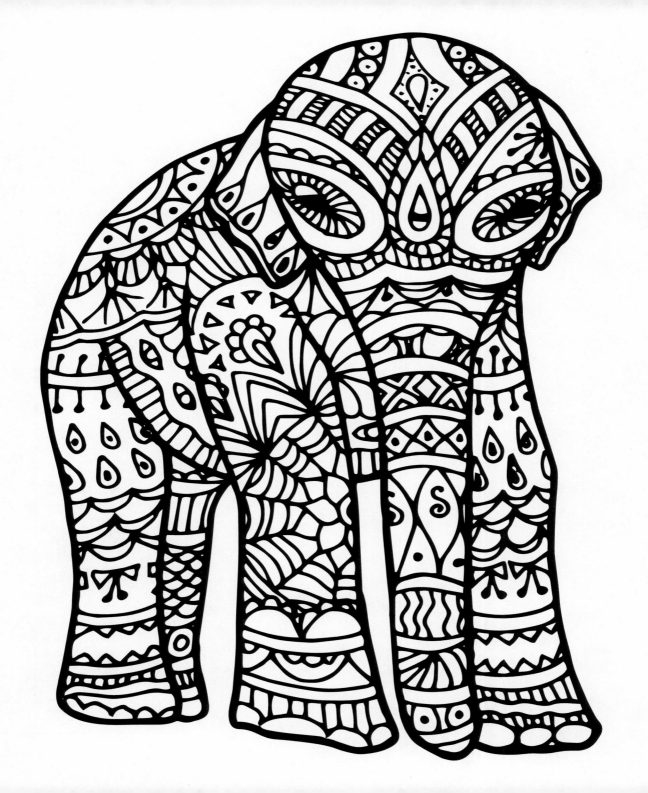

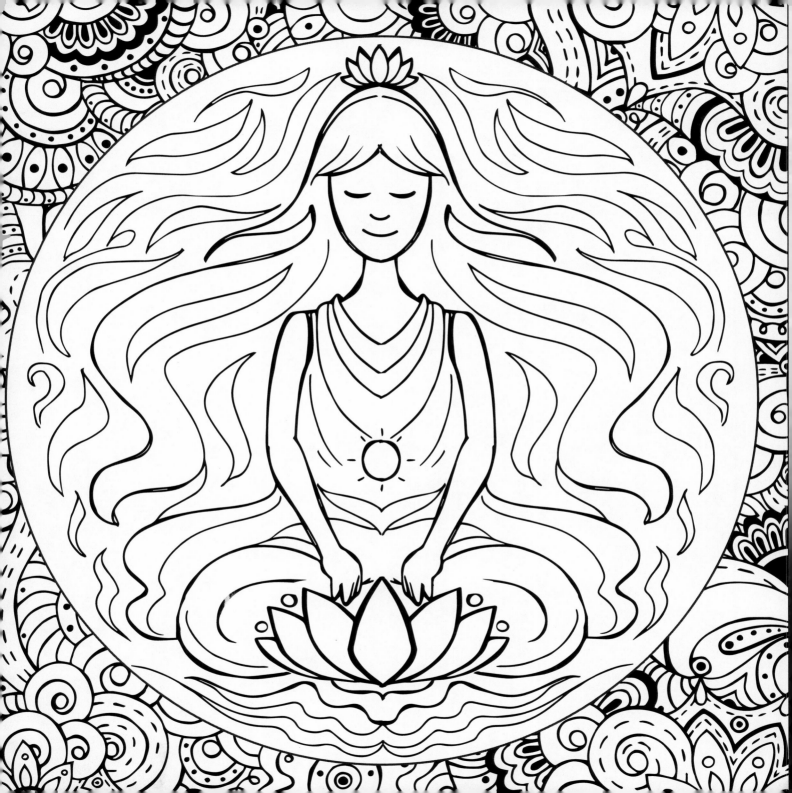

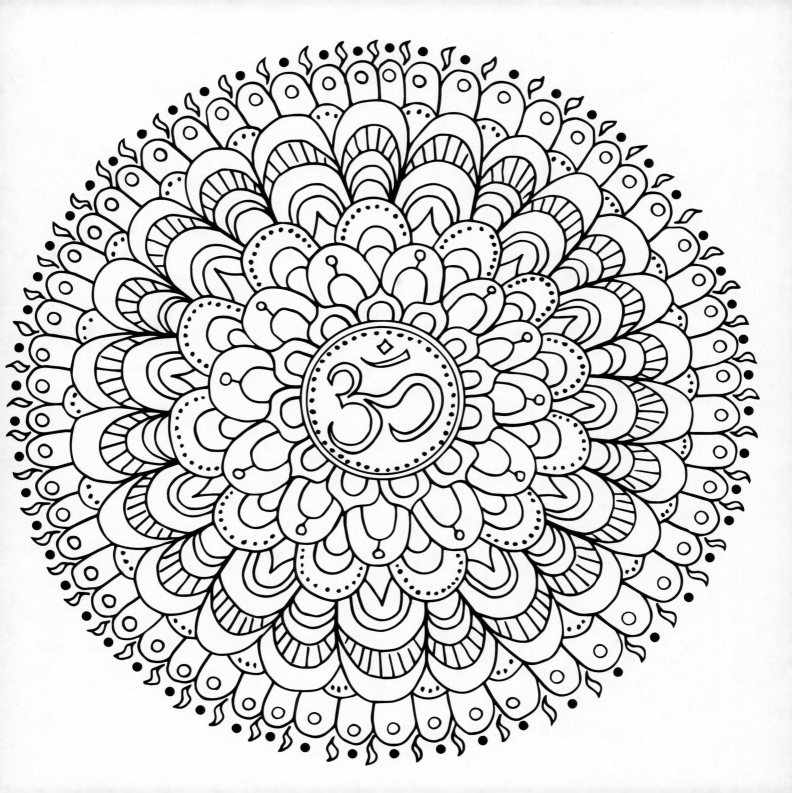

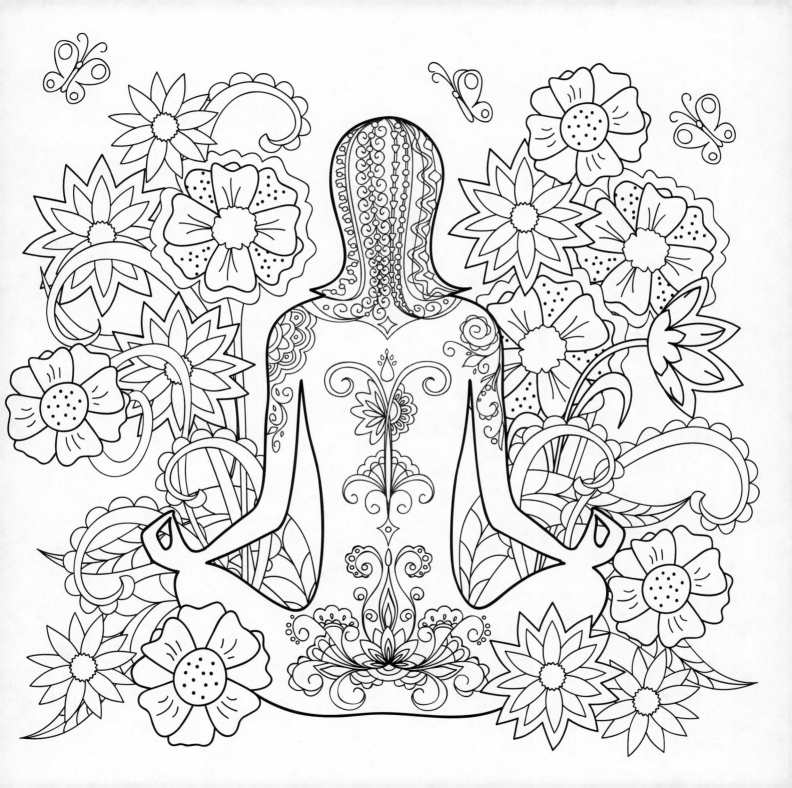

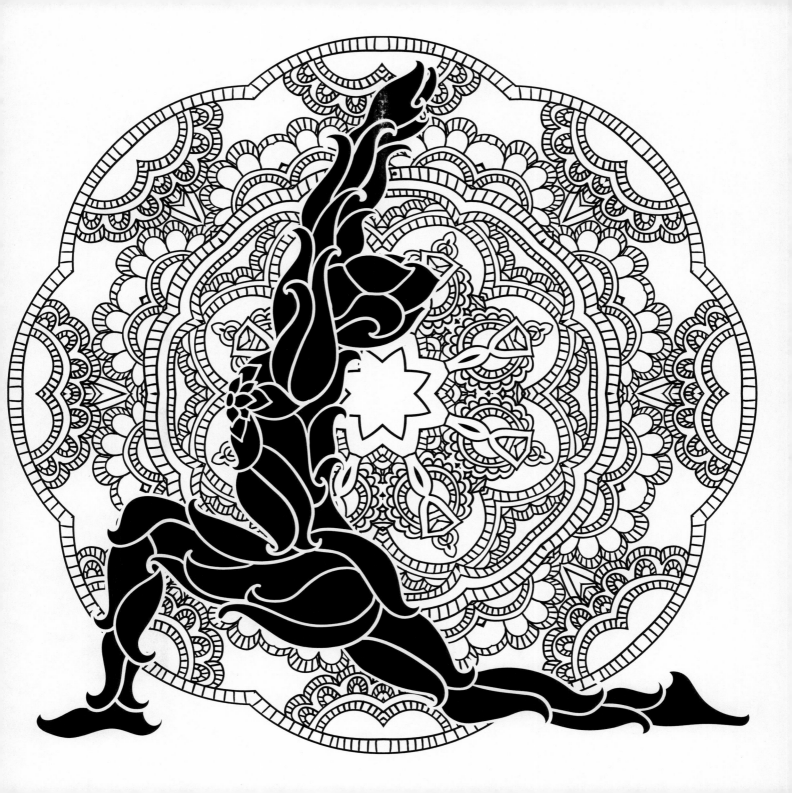

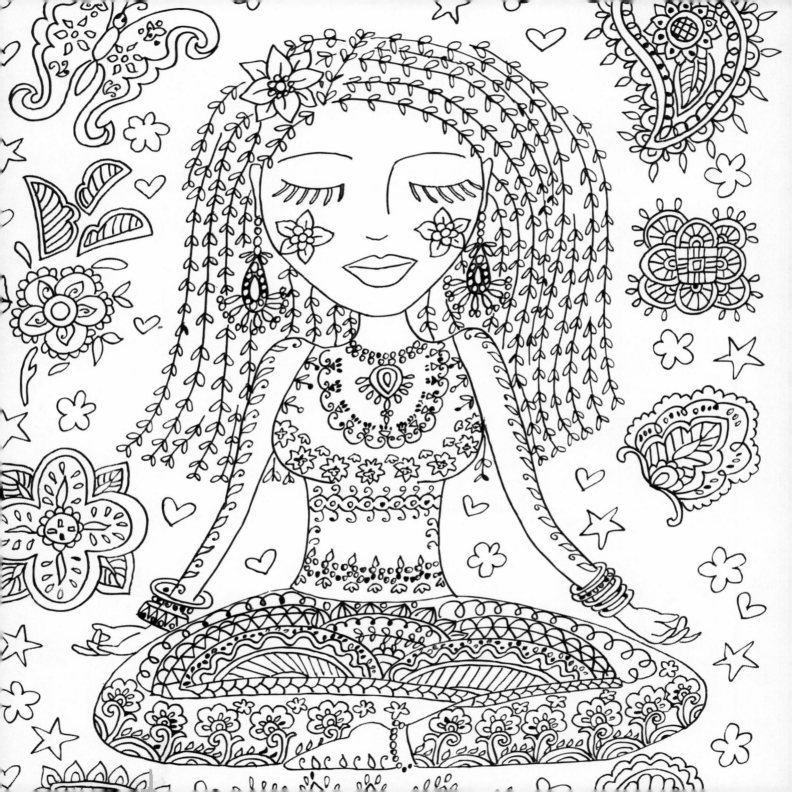

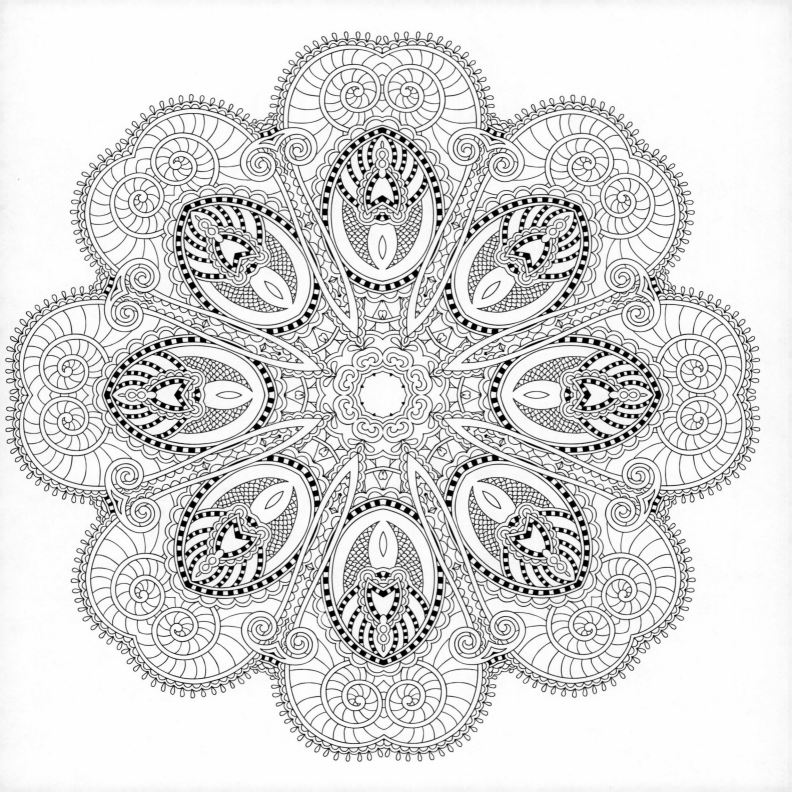

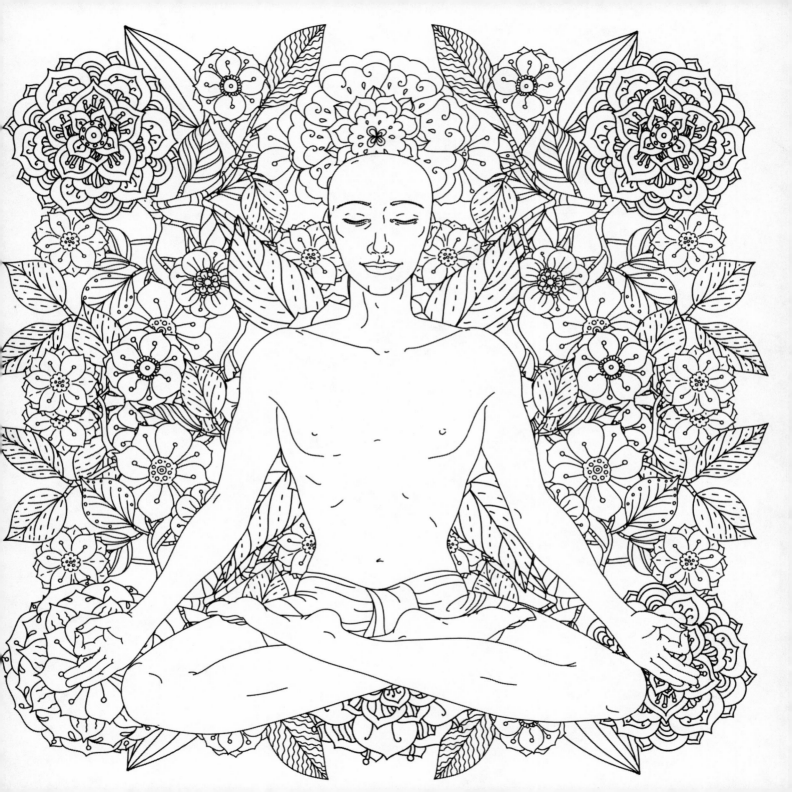

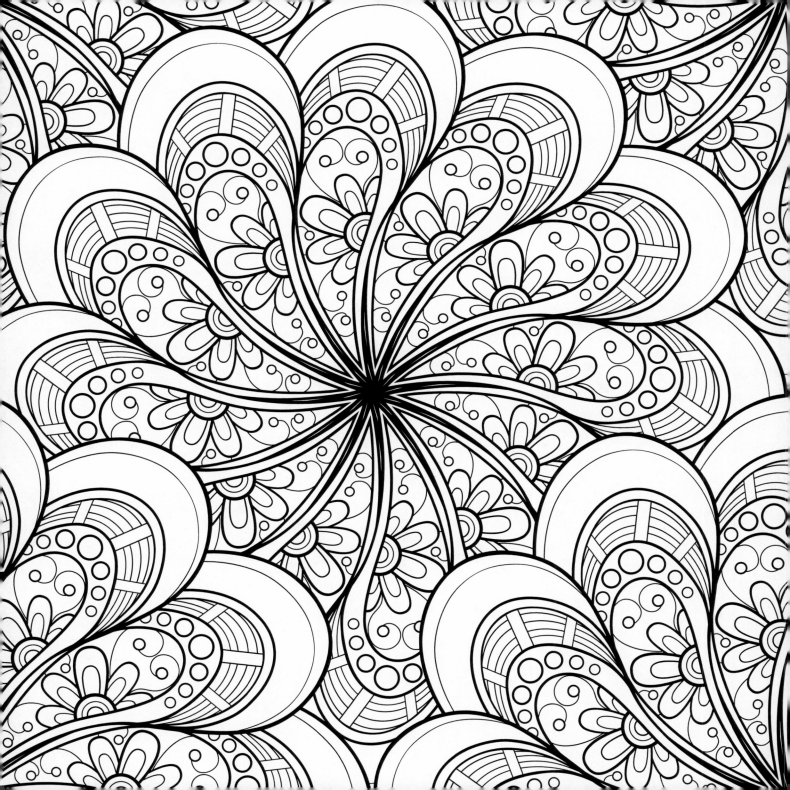

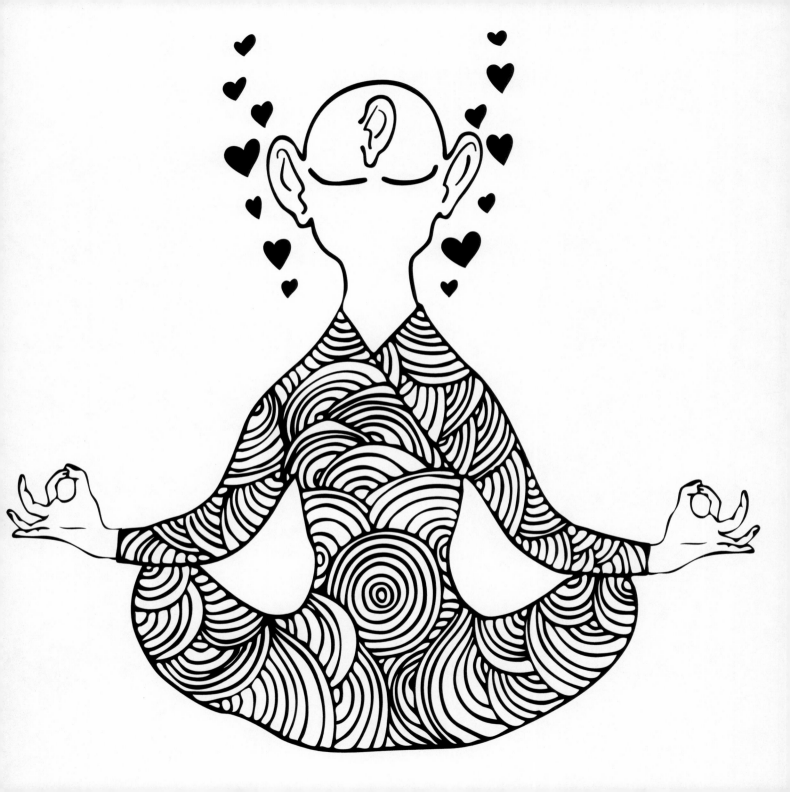

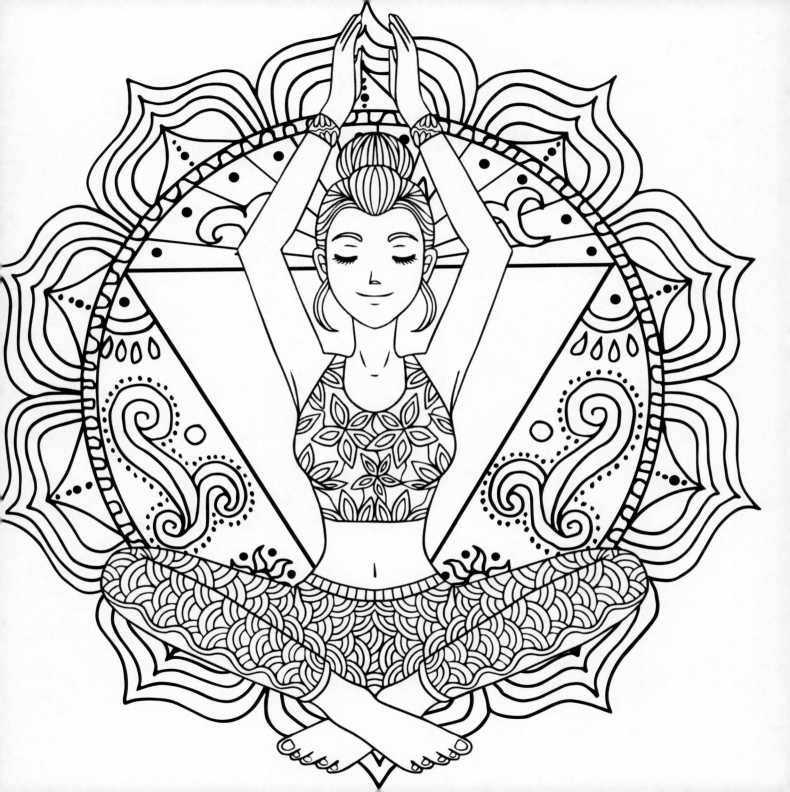

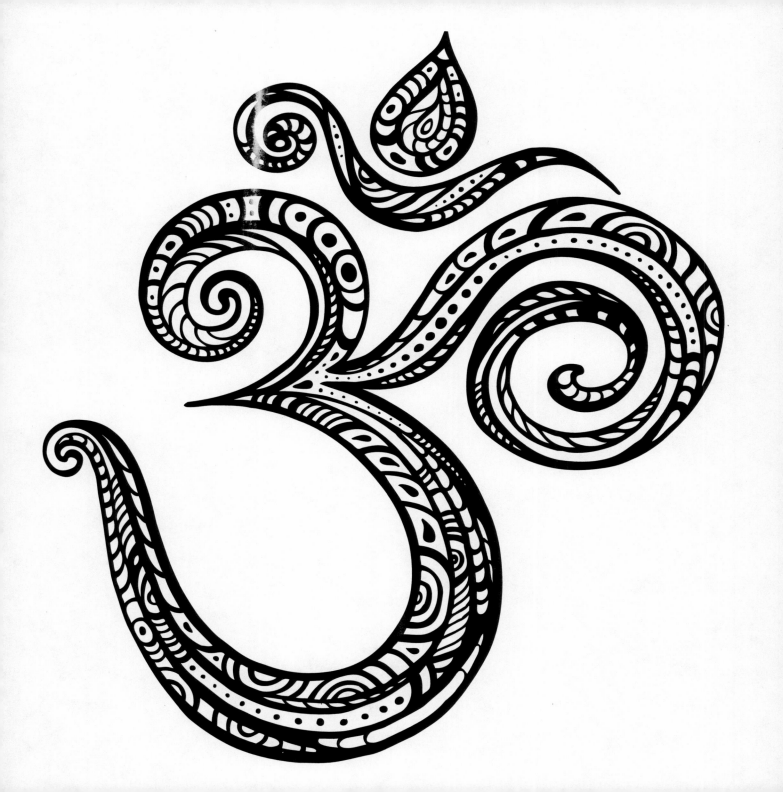

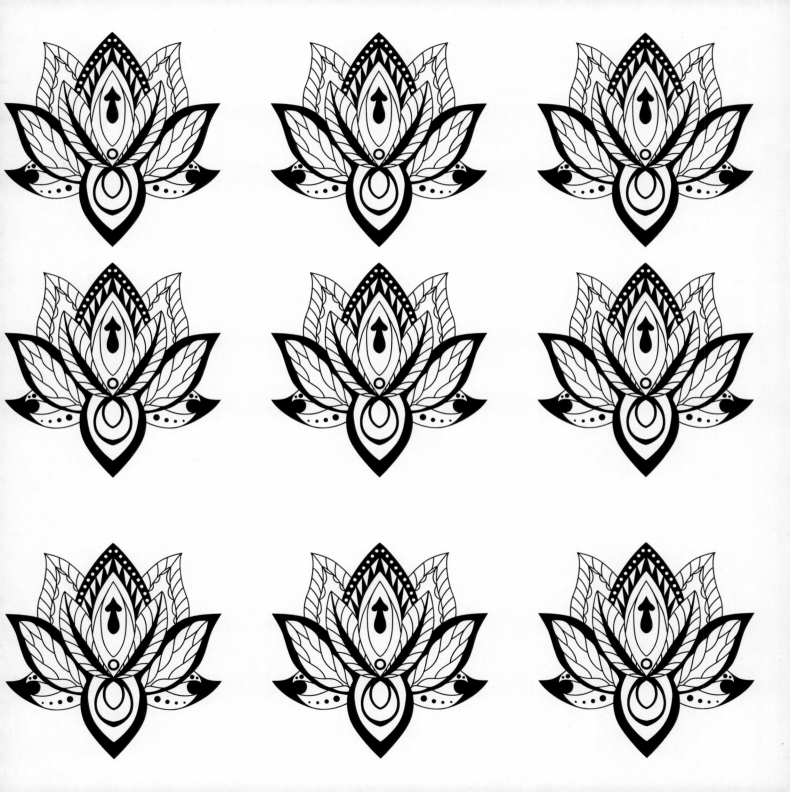

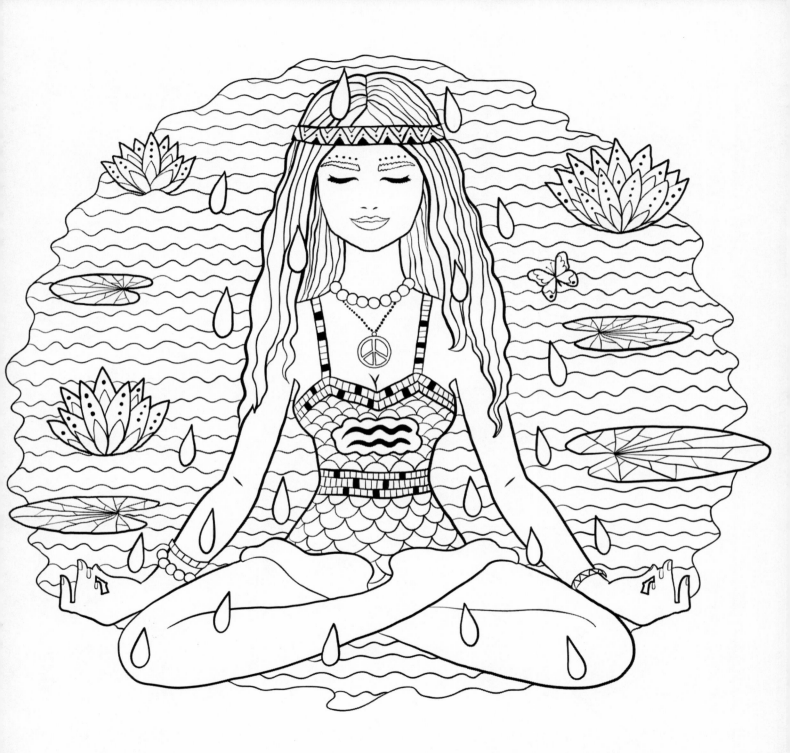

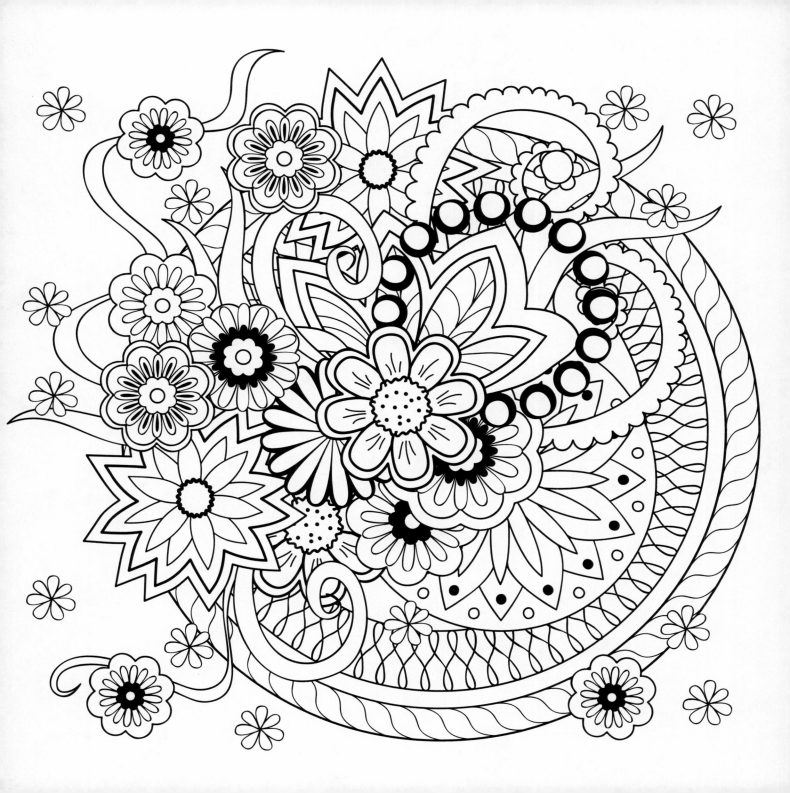

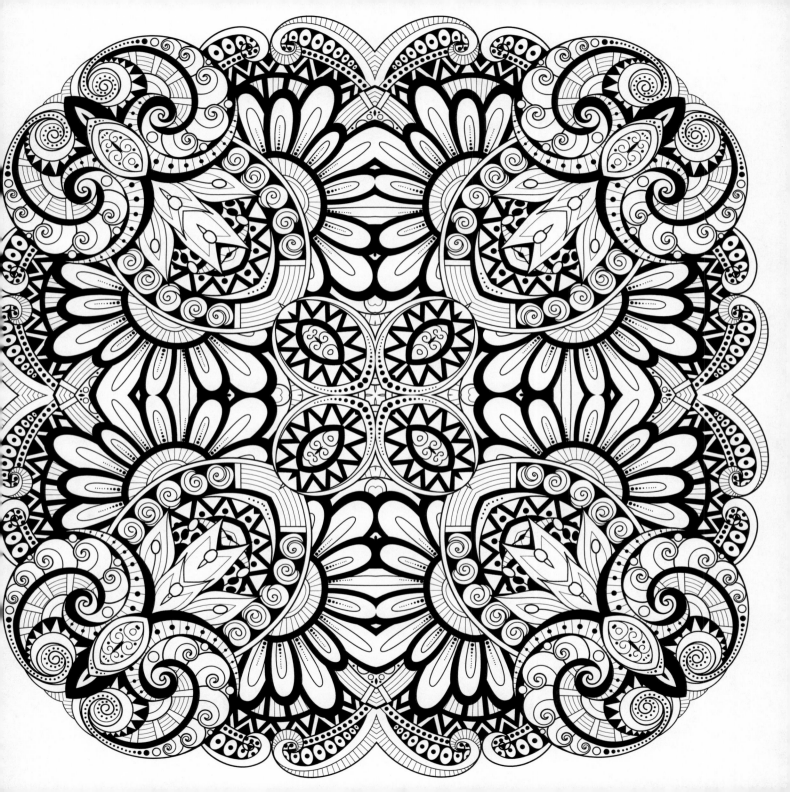

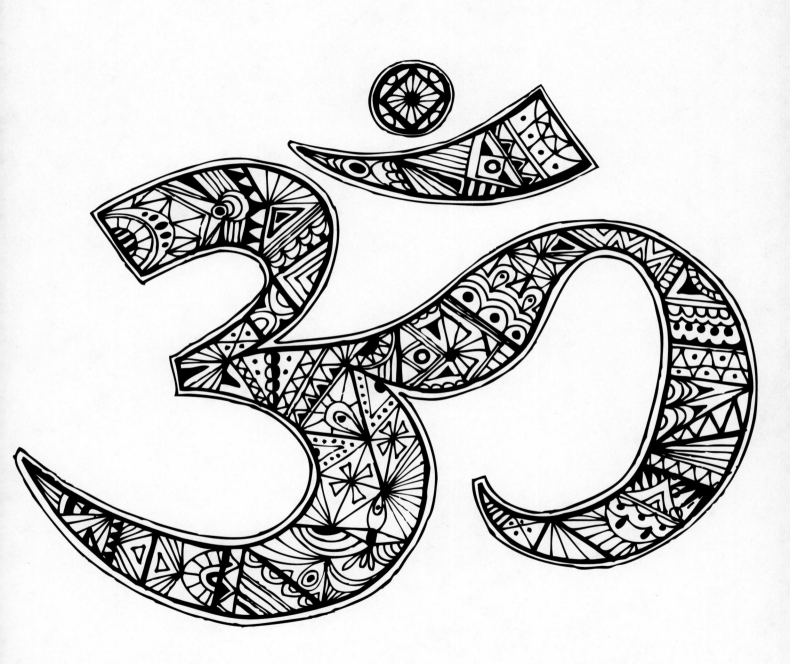

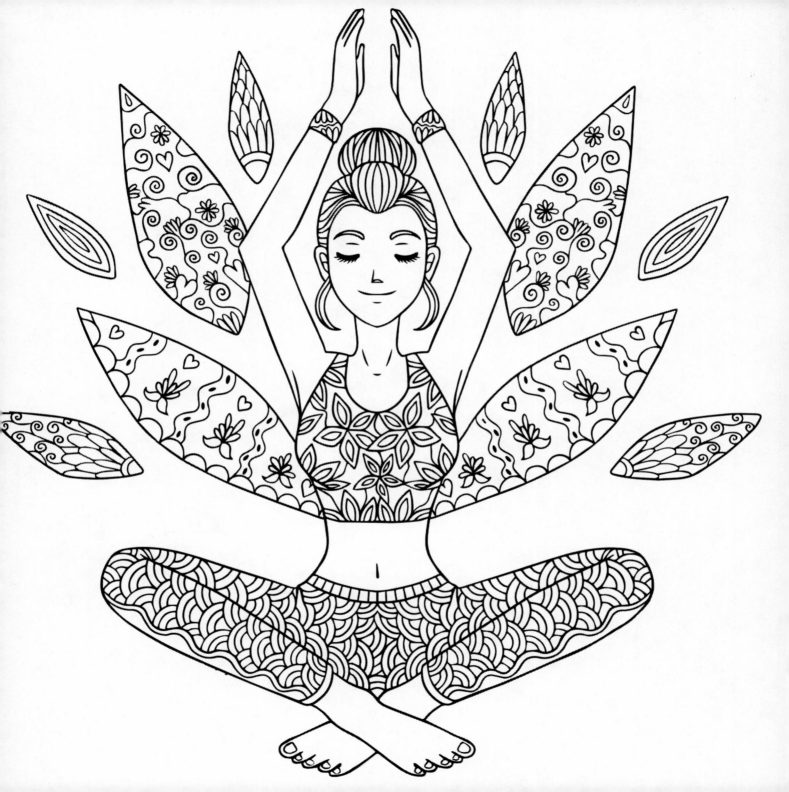

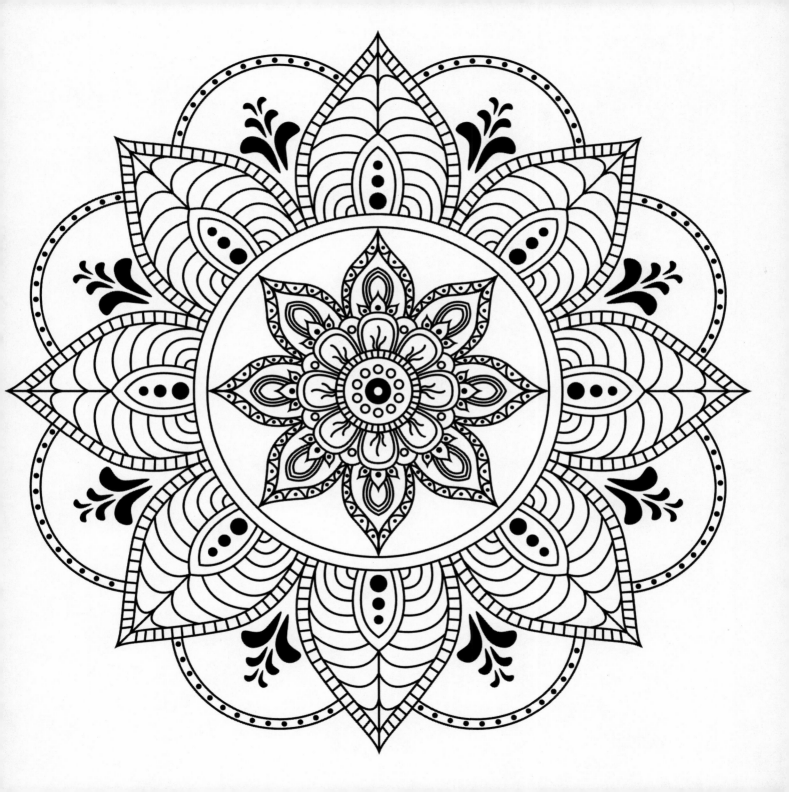

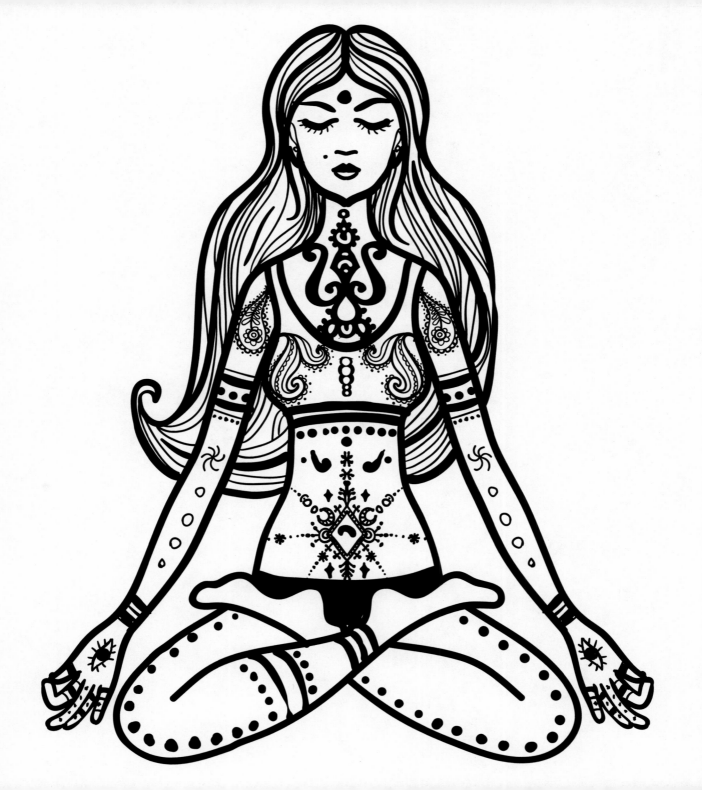

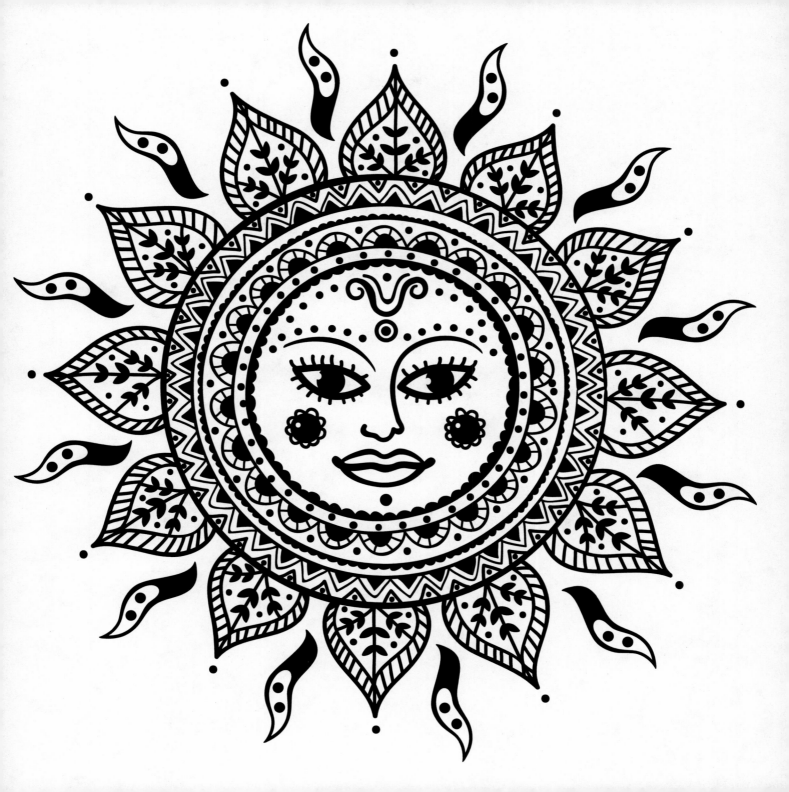

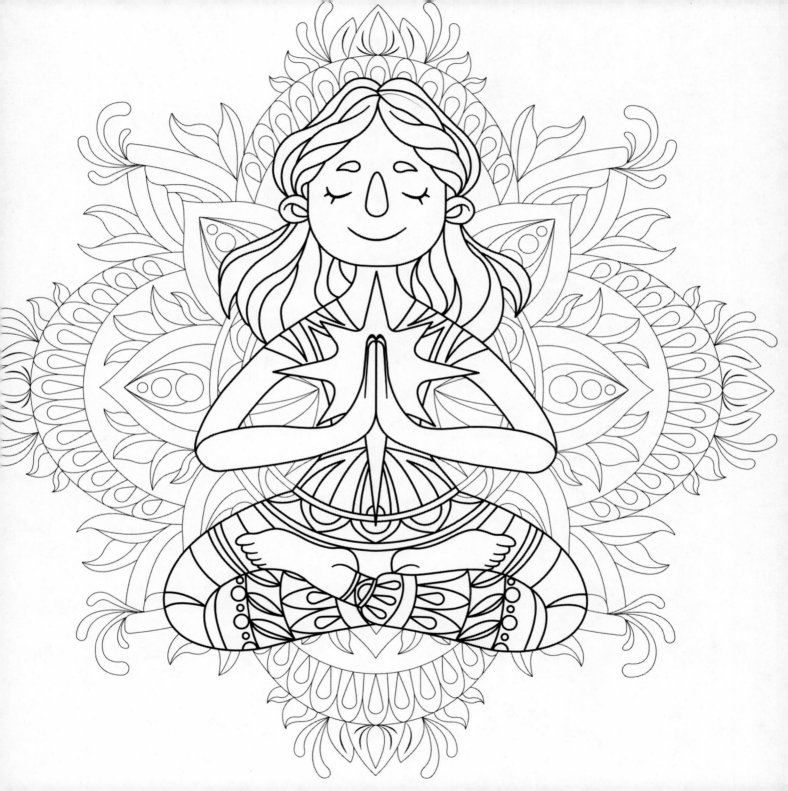

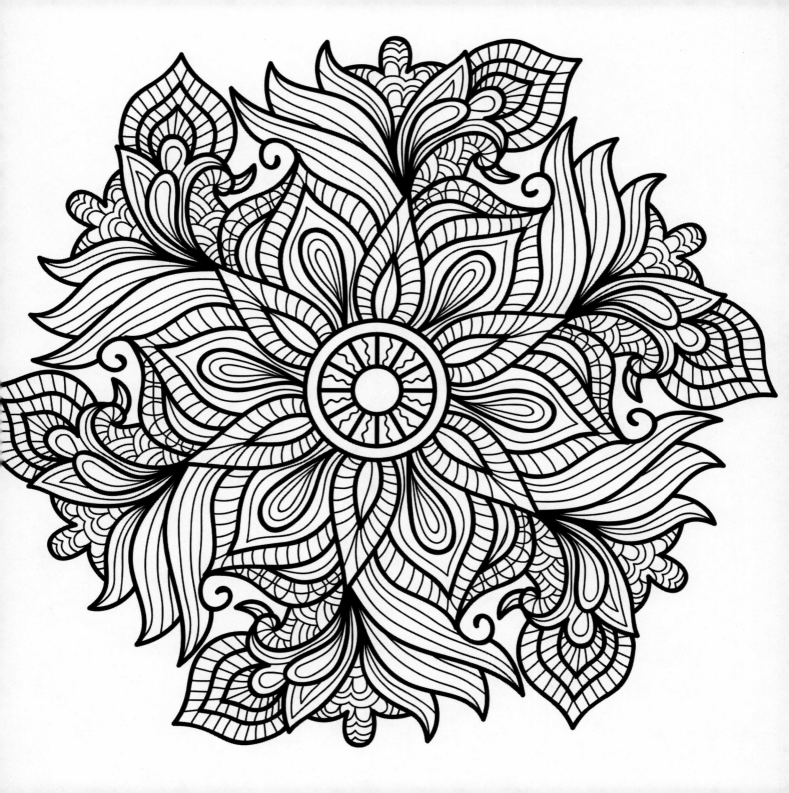

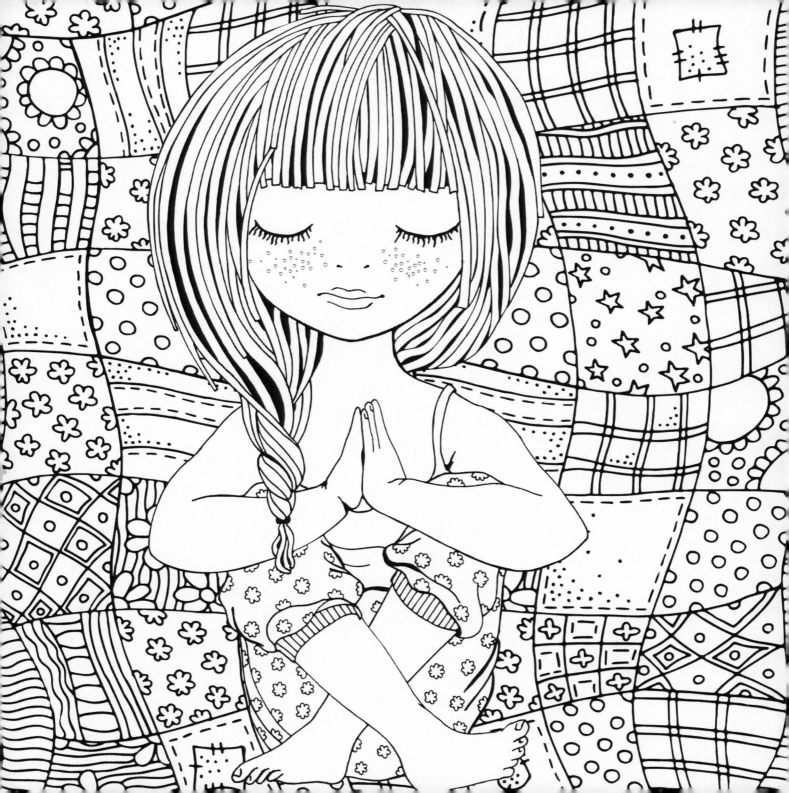

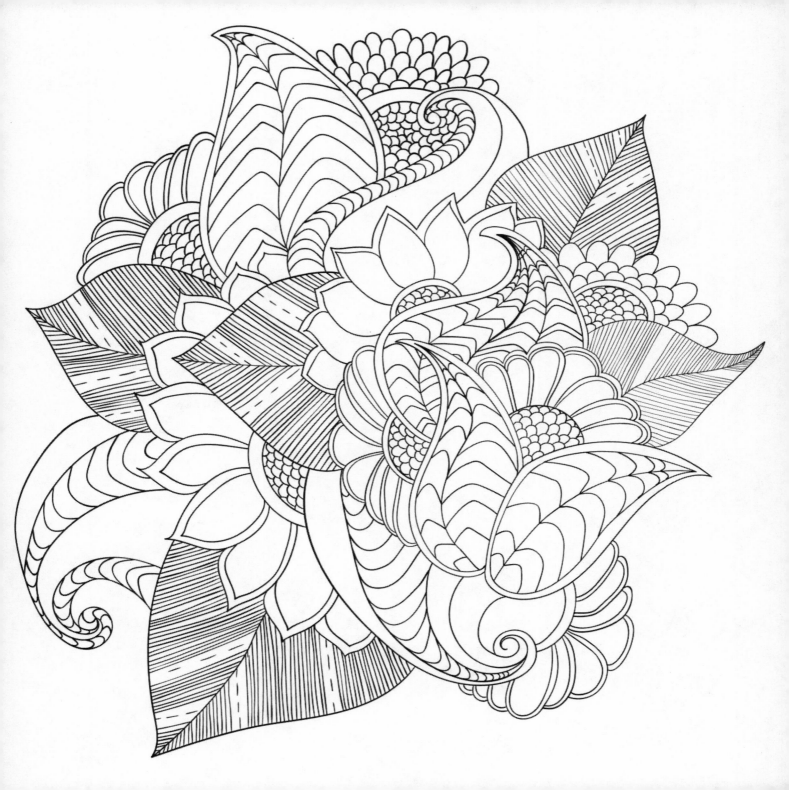

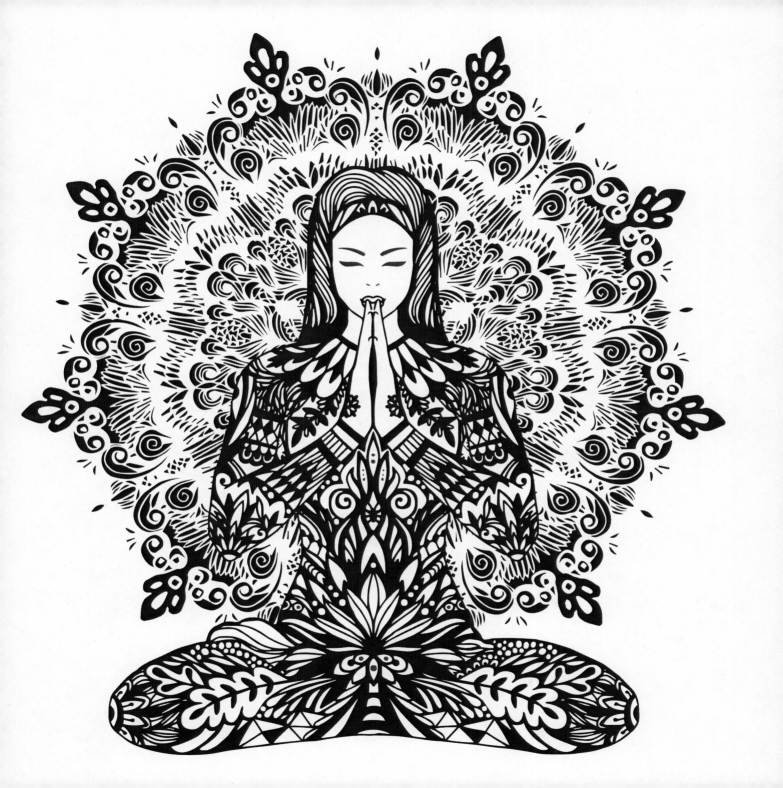

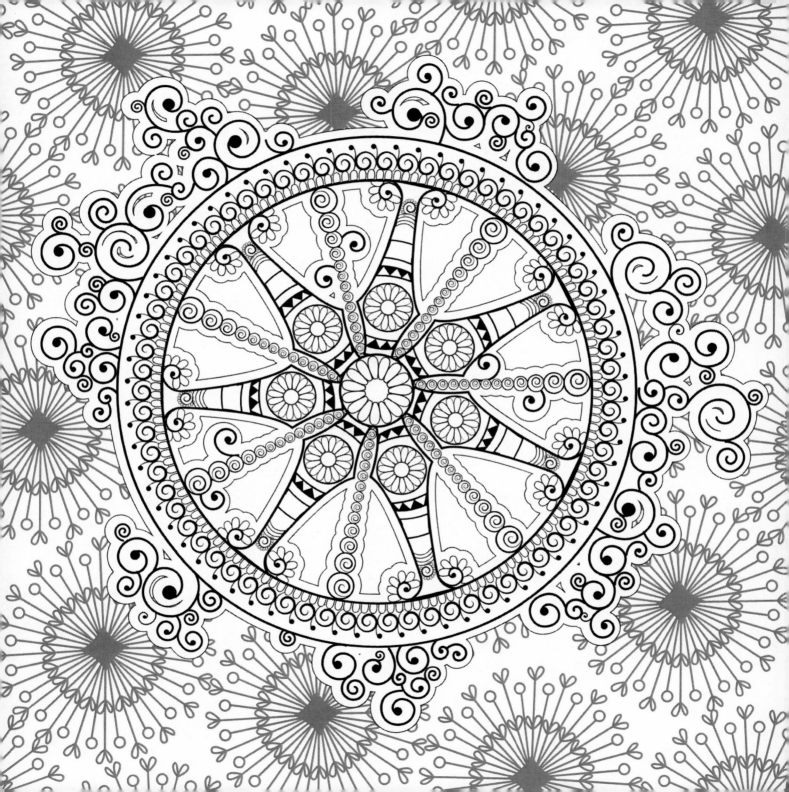

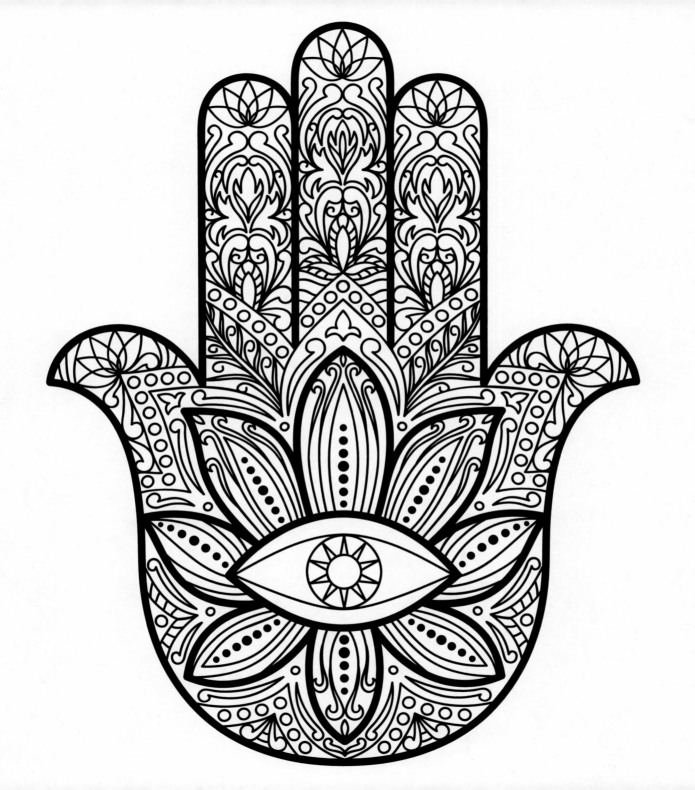

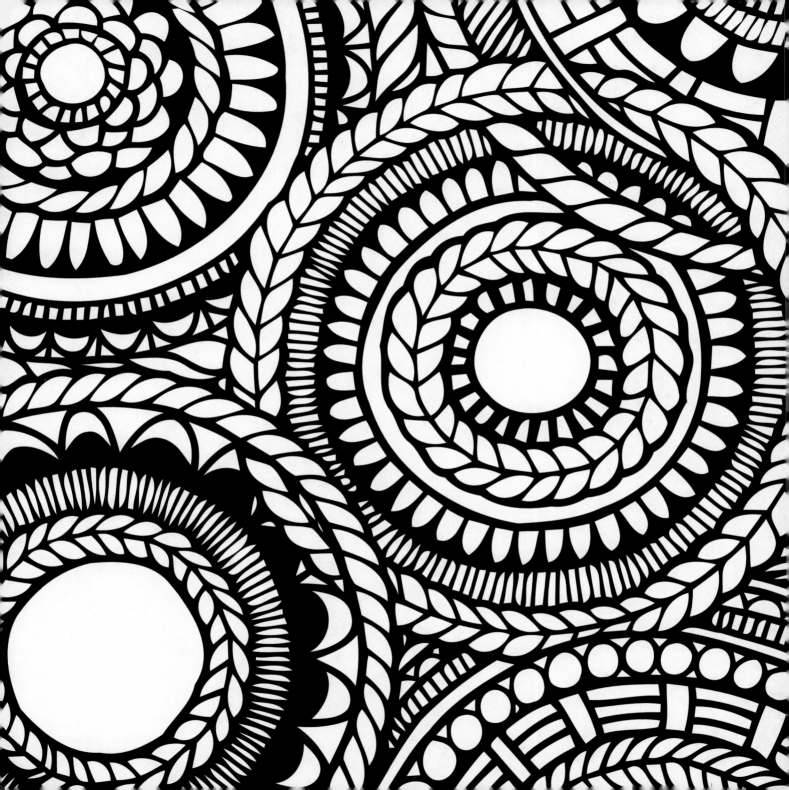

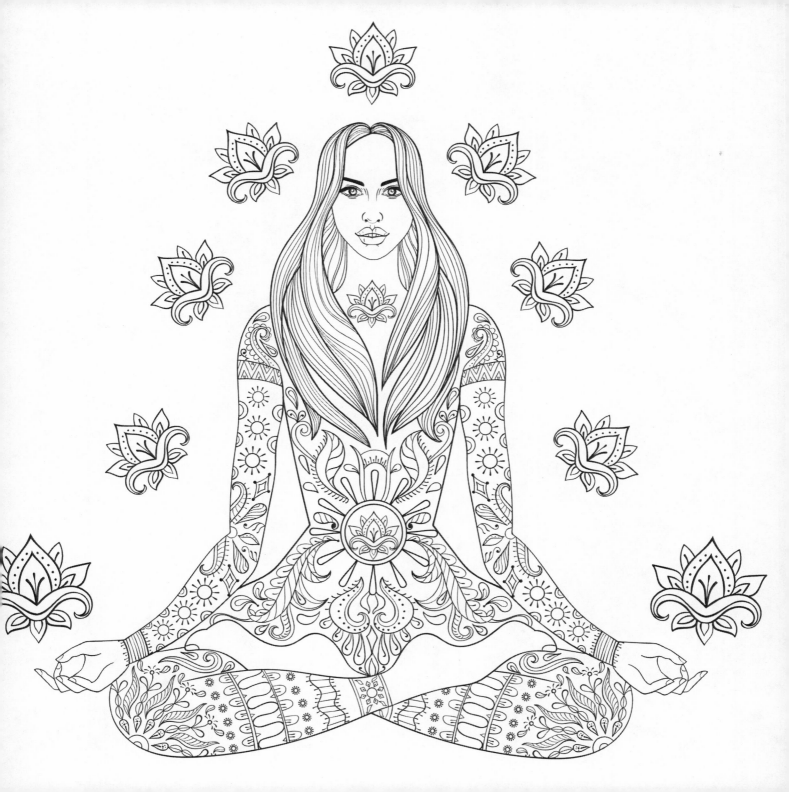

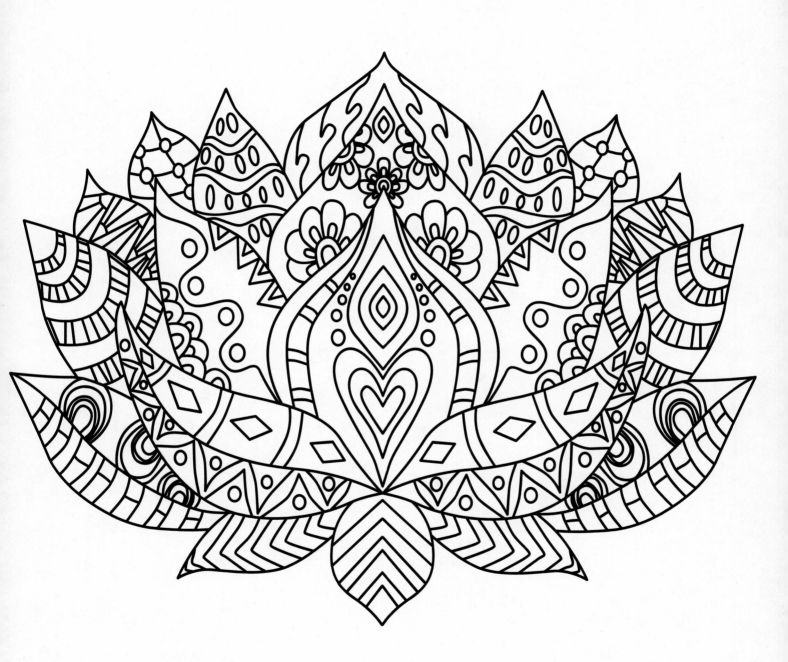

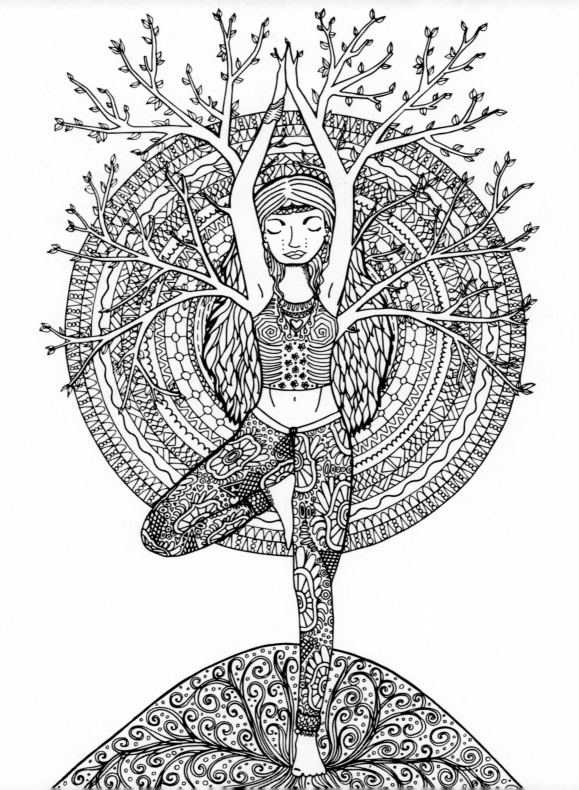

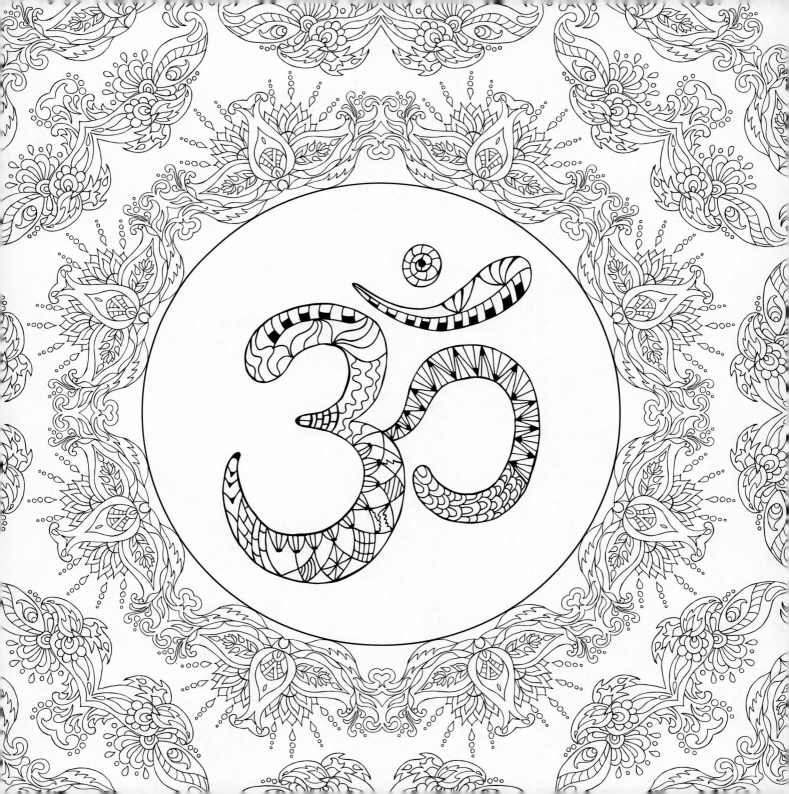

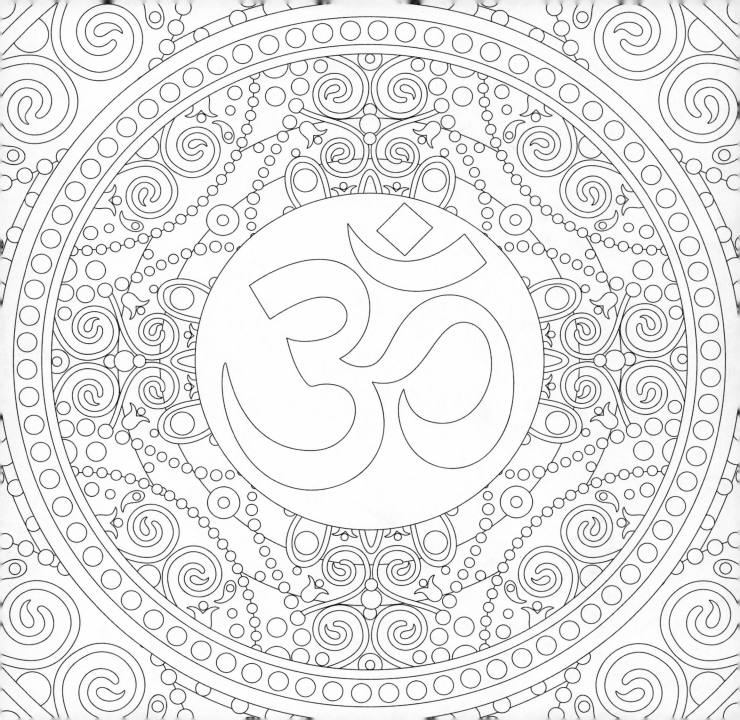

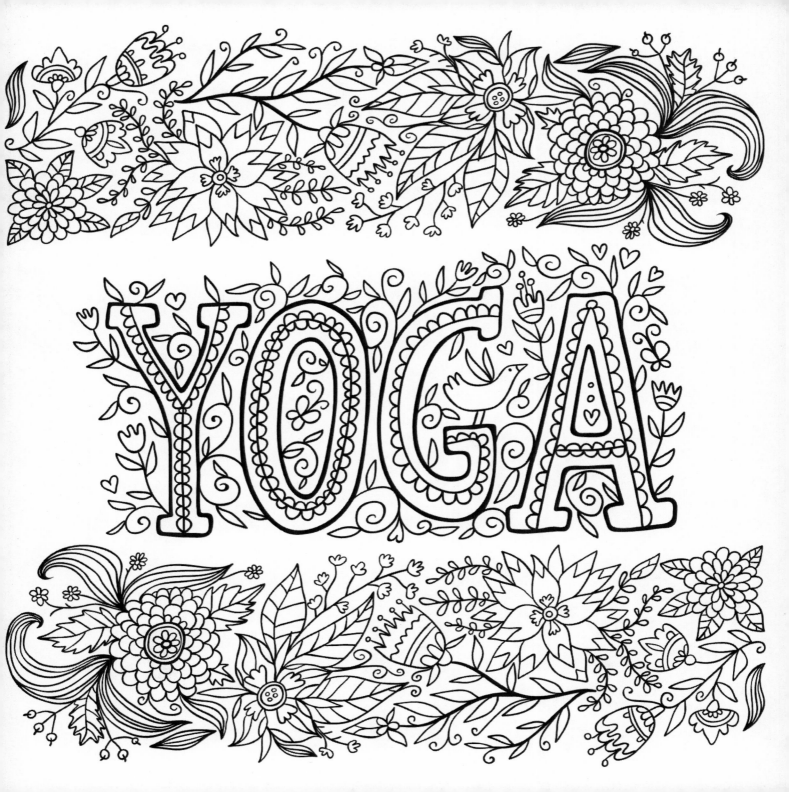

Color Test Page

Other amazing adult coloring books available online at:

CNandJ.com

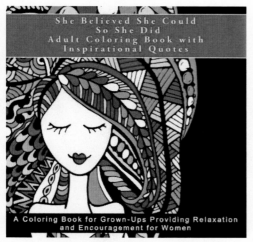

She Believed She Could So She
Did Adult Coloring Book with
Inspirational Quotes

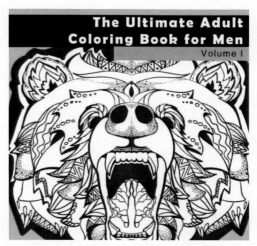

The Ultimate Adult Coloring
Book for Men

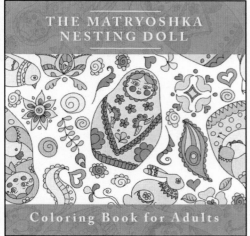

The Matryoshka Nesting Doll
Coloring Book for Adults

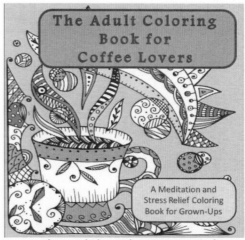

The Adult Coloring Book for
Coffee Lovers